How I Reversed
CONGESTIVE
Heart Failure

Tony Westbrooks

How I Reversed Congestive Heart Failure

Cover & Interior Design by Tony Westbrooks
Interior Format & Layout by Tony Westbrooks

All rights reserved. No part of this book may be reproduced in any form by any electronic or mechanical means including photocopying, recording, or information storage and retrieval without permission in writing from the author.

Copyright © 2017 by Anthony W Westbrooks

ISBN-13: 978-1542429481
ISBN-10: 154242948X

Printed in the USA

Dedicated in the Memory of
Wardell William Westbrooks

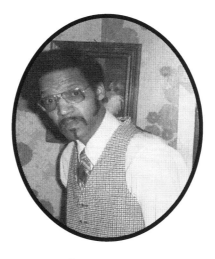

No child no matter of their age can prepare themselves to say goodbye to their father. On September 8, 2012, when I laid my eyes on your lifeless body for the last time, I wish I would have had this conversation with you as a child. If I could rewind time and revisit the first time I sat on your lap, I would say these words to you. "Dad, whatever lifestyle you decide to live will play an instrumental part in how I will live my life, aware of it or not. I appreciate and admire your work ethics and commitment to provide for our family. I'm proud of you dad and the many other fathers who fought for their dignity as men. But there's one fight fathers are losing every day that have a major impact on their families. Dad, were we blind or naive to the seriousness that men in our family died from heart-related issues and strokes? Men in our family as young as 30 years of age suffered from heart complications. We said farewell to three men within a 16 month period. The same fate that took your dad from you, took you from us, came to take me away from mines. As if it was yesterday, I remember seeing you sitting up in your hospital bed a few days before your departure from us. You made this statement; "I wish there were more I could have left for my kids." Dad, I never imagine that three years later, I would be sitting in that same hospital bed, with the same medical condition, making the same statement. There I realized what your children wanted from you, is what my kids want from me. That is a healthy father who will be around to share in their family's lives. I turned my back to fate and decided to fight not knowing the outcome. I owe it to God, myself, my kids, your dad and the men in our family who passed away from this condition. Dad, I apologize for not knowing then what I know now, that I may have been able to help you through this.

So here we are, and nothing I can do or say will change your situation. At my best, I promise Dad to be a blessing to our family and to those who may be feeling the hopelessness you felt as a result of this condition."

We miss you Pops

CONTENTS:

1. My Life before Congestive Heart Failure   **5**

- Warning signs
- Symptoms that sent me to the ER

2. What I've learned about Congestive Heart Failure   **11**

- What is Congestive Heart Failure
- What is ejection fractions

3. Life Changing Steps I Took to Control My Congestive Heart Failure   **15**

- The importance of checking vitals
- The importance of a low sodium diet
- How to approach a low sodium diet
- High blood pressure and your heart
- A healthy alternative to Lower high blood pressure
- Restoring erectile function

4. Don't Be Afraid to Exercise   **35**

- It's never too late to exercise
- CHF may improve with exercise
- Effect of exercise are not age-dependent
- Easy type of workouts for CHF patients

5. Developed a Healthy Mindset and Remain Focused   **43**

6. Minimize the Risk as a Commercial Driver   **51**

- Why Positive attitude may bring longer life

- Become excited about improving your condition

7. Conclusions   61

- Don't Label Your Condition for Failure

8. Low Sodium Recipes   65

- Heart Healthy Beet Juice
- Slow Cooker Low Sodium Chili
- Low Sodium Cream of Broccoli Soup
- Kale Chips
- Low Sodium Lemon Pepper Chicken
- Spicy Stuffed Bell Peppers
- Low Sodom Black Eye Peas
- Blackened Red Snapper
- Stuffed Spinach & Crab Mushrooms
- Slow Cooker Falling off the Bone
  Baby Backs Ribs
- Salisbury Steak
- Spicy Jamaican Jerk Hot Wings
- Slow Cooker Spicy Mustard Greens with Kale

Life Vitals Daily Log Sheet   77

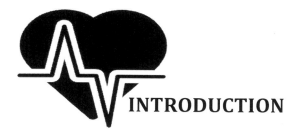

INTRODUCTION

I'm not a medical physician nor do I have extensive education on heart disease or congestive heart failure (CHF). I'm simply your everyday guy who found himself with a critical medical condition that if not treated correctly, could easily cost me my life. Congestive Heart Failure is a severe condition that shouldn't ever be ignored. Honestly, I can say when I was first informed of my situation; I wasn't concerned about who else was suffering from this condition or other people's opinions. What was fresh in my mind was three years prior my father was diagnosed with CHF and died four months later. So you can understand my concern.

On May 18, 2015, at 11:30 pm, I found myself in a hospital bed in the ER from what I the thought was fatigue. An ER doctor came alongside my bed and informed me that my heart was very weak and test results indicated that I was suffering from Congestive Heart Failure. BAM! Now I knew how Wile E. Coyote felt when he ran smack into a painted brick wall he thought was an open tunnel while chasing the Roadrunner. For the first time in my life, I felt completely helpless. I've never heard anything positive about congestive heart failure, and the majority of all whom I've talked with about it, other than medical personnel had a family member or knew someone who died from this illness. "What's next" was the difficult question I had to address. I knew I couldn't deny my situation, but did that mean do nothing? Allow fate to determine my destiny? I've witnessed this way of thinking with my dad and so many others diagnosed with CHF.

"It doesn't matter what happened to you, what matters is what you are going to do about it. You're going to have to make a declaration that you are going to stand up for peace of mind;"

Les Brown, motivational speaker

I've been here before, and this isn't my first rodeo overcoming severe health issues. December of 1999, I had open heart surgery to repair my Mitral Valve. My Mitral Valve wasn't replaced. Instead, an Annuloplasty Ring was placed in my valve to resize the opening.

My surgeon instructed me following the surgery that my physical activities would be limited, and my Mitral Value would most likely have to be replaced within seven years. Seventeen years later, I've competed in several Natural Bodybuilding Competitions, 5K races, and four Spartan Races. To this date, all of my test results show a strong, healthy heart and my mitral valve have remained healthy.

I know firsthand what a person experiences when they are first diagnosed with CHF. I'm more excited today writing this book than the day I decided to take control of my congestive heart failure. My objective with this book is not only to encourage you but also to share with you the steps I took to improve my CHF. Six months after being diagnosed with CHF and making significant life changes, I received a surprising phone call from the Registered Nurse (RN) who was responsible for monitoring my progress. She called me after my second Echo Heart Scan test result, and stated,

"Mr. Westbrooks, I'm not sure what happened, but I'm happy to inform you that the Echocardiogram test result shows that your heart's ejection fraction improved tremendous, you're no longer considered a CHF patient.

What do you say? Let's start the healing process.

"Let us not become weary in doing good, for at the proper time we will reap a harvest if we do not give up." Galatians 6:9

CHAPTER 1

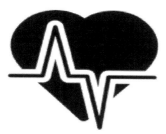

My Life before Congestive Heart Failure and Warning Signs

I lived a pretty healthy life before being diagnosed with Congestive Heart Failure. Before this, the only serious health condition I encountered was having open heart surgery 15 years earlier to repair my Mitral Valve which consisted of an Annuloplasty Ring being placed in the valve and controlling my Hypertension. I remember after my open heart surgery, my surgeon instructing me that I would not be able to return to the fitness level I was at before the surgery. He felt it would be safer if I didn't lift any weights heavier than 150LB. At age 39, this was a major setback to my way of thinking, and I struggled mentally with what type of quality of life I would be living from here on out? There's something magical about the mind of the youthful; that gung-ho "I can do this" drive they have. I took this state of mind, and I started reading everything I could about CHF and how to live with it. I was so persistent about surviving and improving my health that my diet was on point, I modified my fitness workout, and begin studying to become a certified Personal Fitness Trainer. Three years after open heart surgery I was in such good physical condition that I started competing as a Natural Bodybuilder. I wasn't one of the big guys, just lean with a good symmetry. I was falling in love with my new lifestyle, and because of my passion for remaining healthy, I had no problem staying disciplined. Then comes the shock of feeling unmatched in the title fight, the challenger, Congestive Heart Failure. Who would have ever thought that Mr. Fitness, Tony Westbrooks, would be challenged with congestive heart failure? I still remember that night I laid in a hospital bed in the ER. Let me take you back before this event; I knew something was going on with my health, but I couldn't place my finger on it. I just figured I was out of shape or just getting too old for certain exercises. One major symptom I was experiencing was fatigue. It didn't take much exercise to cause me to feel exhausted and as time went on my exhaustion escalated. I found myself avoiding lower body exercises because it took so much out of me. When I would try to do strength exercises like deadlifts, leg presses or bench presses, my left foot would become numb, and I would begin feeling tightness in the left side of my chest.

I started associating my symptoms to overworking and modified my workouts to something lighter. I know it doesn't make any sense that I didn't make an appointment to speak with my primary physician. Another symptom I was experiencing that was very disturbing was an irregular heartbeat known as Arrhythmia. Now if you ever experienced irregular heartbeats, (Arrhythmia), you know firsthand, it's a scary feeling. The first thought to come to mind is that you're having a "Heart Attack." I would usually experience these irregular heartbeats during periods of rest, like relaxing, sitting up or lying in bed. I would never get these irregular heartbeats while exerting energy or exercising. I went to the ER several times for these irregular heartbeats, and a Heart attack was ruled out, so I begin to ignore the symptom and dealt with them as they came on me.

Other symptoms at the time although I didn't know they were symptoms were light-headiness, bloated adnominal feeling and constipation. It wasn't until one night at work I came to the realization that enough was enough. The symptoms were starting to overtake me, and I felt like I could no longer operate normally. My health was at a crucial point, and I didn't realize the seriousness of my symptoms.

I can't tell you how grateful I am how God looks over our wellbeing when we're not aware of our circumstances, even in my stubbornness. My daughter who at the time was in her last semester at UC Davis Medical School just happened to call me to see how I was doing. She could tell in my voice that I wasn't feeling well. I shared with her the symptoms I was experiencing, and she said to me, "Dad, I think you're experiencing Congestive Heart Failure. You need to go to the ER right away." I responded by telling her I would, knowing I had four hours left on my shift and planned on going to the ER after work. I can't stress to you how painful the next four hours of work were for me trying to operate a 40-foot bus under those symptoms. With my symptoms escalating, and not addressing it by going to the ER, I was placing my health and the lives of others in jeopardy by pushing the limits. When I got off work that evening, I told myself that if I was to go directly home and lay down, there was a good possibility I wouldn't be alive in the morning. That's how awful I felt. So I made my way to the ER, and I explained to the registration attendant my symptoms, that I was a heart patient because of my previous open heart surgery. They immediately took my blood pressure reading and based on the register nurses expression; I knew it couldn't have been good reading. She called to another nurse for a second opinion, and the ER Doctor suggested taking an echocardiography reading. This time when the nurse read the results from the echocardiography, she sprinted out of the room and before you know it I was lying in a hospital bed, hospital gown, iv and hooked to a hospital monitor. Several hours later an ER doctor came in and explained that the test results indicated that my heart was fragile and I was showing signs of Congestive Heart Failure, and I came in with a blood pressure reading of 198/139. He went on to say, "Mr. Westbrooks it looks like you will be with us for a few days." During my hospital stay, a lot of information was given to me, because of my lack of understanding and the shock of my condition; I couldn't comprehend most of it. Seven days later I returned to work with a doctor's note only to encounter my second obstacle. Word had gotten back to my employer that I had been hospitalized for a heart-related issue. Because I was a commercial driver, my employer was concerned about the safety of the passengers and the company vehicle. I was placed on administrative leave until I could be seen by the company's Medical Physician and considered fit for duty again. Can you believe that this entire process to return to work took six months? But now I see God's hand in all of this because it was a life-changing experience and the inspiration for writing this book.

"Many of life's failures are people who did not realize how close they were to success when they gave up."
Thomas Edison

CHAPTER 2

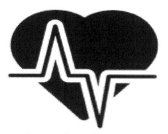

What I've learned about Congestive Heart Failure

To learn that you have Congestive Heart Failure is one of the most shocking news someone could ever hear. I'm not talking about having a common cold or the flu bug, something that you could purchase over the counter medication for or ride it out, I'm talking about the heart, a major organ in the body. What I've come to learn with myself, and with many others who have congestive heart failure, is that fear comes because of our lack of knowledge of the disease. It took doing research on my part to realize not everyone dies from congestive heart failure and that there are different types of CHF. The broken record that was playing in my mind was that my father had died from CHF four months after being diagnosed. My dad had other contributing health issues like Chronic Obstructive Pulmonary Disease (COPD), and he made no attempts to change his sodium/salt intake, which placed more strain on his failing heart. This motivated me to learn all I could about this disease.

What is Congestive Heart Failure? Congestive Heart Failure doesn't mean your heart is not working, rather that the heart pumping power is weaker than normal. With Congestive Heart Failure, blood moves through the heart and body at a slower rate, causing pressure in the heart to increase. As a result, the heart cannot pump enough oxygen and nutrients to meet the body's need. The chambers of the heart respond by stretching to hold more blood to pump through the body, referred to as Heart Failure Enlarging. Enabling the heart to contract more forcefully, helping pump more blood. This helps the blood to keep moving, but the heart muscle walls may eventually weaken and become unable to pump as efficiently. As a result, the kidneys may respond by causing the body to retain fluids (water) and salt. If fluids build up in the arms, legs, ankles, feet, lungs, or other organs, the body becomes congested and Congestive Heart Failure is the term used to describe this condition.

To put is simply, CHF means the heart isn't pumping blood as well as it once did. It's no longer delivering all the blood and oxygen that the body and organs need to work normally. In turn, can make some physical activities more challenging, even everyday things you use to do without a second thought. I believe one vital piece of information every CHF patient needs to know about is their heart ejection fraction number.

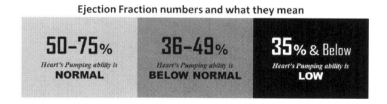

As I mentioned earlier, my father died from congestive heart failure. I witnessed his heart weakening, swelling of his legs, oxygen tanks, and part of his heart dying which led to kidney failure; all took place within a period of four months. It seemed that just about everyone I talked with about my condition had a family member or knew someone who died from congestive heart failure, pushing me into a deeper depression. Studies show that many diagnosed with a life-threatening disease may experience four emotional stages: shock, fear, anger, and acceptance. I can say I experienced all four but decided to add a fifth stage -IMPROVEMENT. When I thought about my family, my two beautiful granddaughters whose lives I desired to be a part of, I decided to fight for my life. Not only for me, but also for those who cared about and loved me. God forbid, but if I was going to die from congestive heart failure, I wanted my children and grandchildren to remember that their dad and papa fought the good fight for a better quality of life.

"Failure is only the opportunity to begin again, this time more intelligently."
Henry Ford

CHAPTER 3

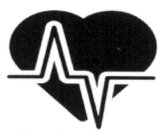

Life Changing Steps I Took to Control My Congestive Heart Failure

The Importance of Checking Vitals. Ok, you have congestive heart failure, so where do you start? There's a wealth of information available, but how do you make it relevant to where you are? You may have felt overwhelmed because of the severity of the illness, so much so that you question if it's too late to do anything that would make a difference. I too pondered these questions within my mind and felt handicapped because I didn't know where to start. I was privileged to have a health care provider that offered a monitoring program for those newly diagnosed with CHF. It provided a guide that created discipline in the area of daily of monitoring of my vitals.

My health care provider even sent an RN to my home to set up a blue tooth vitals monitoring system. The monitoring system consisted of a 7" tablet, finger oximeter, digital scale, and blood pressure monitor. The system would come on each morning with an activated voice saying, "Good Morning, it's time to take your vitals." Seven days a week at 8:00 am consistent. The program on the tablet would guide me through the process, and the readings were sent directly to a nurse practitioner who would contact me within an hour if there was any concern with my vitals. I recall receiving calls within minutes; either to make a change in my medication or to consult on how to reduce my fluid retention. This program helped me to recognize unnoticeable changes in my conditions that I wouldn't have otherwise caught. I remember my body weight going up eight pounds within three days due to fluid retention and as result adjustments were made to my Lasix dosage. This monitoring system program taught me the importance of monitoring your vitals daily or at least several times a week. It wasn't easy at the beginning of this program. Many mornings I found it to be an annoyance and I didn't always want to get up at 8:00 am and take my vitals. I would have to wait until I went through the process of checking my vitals before leaving the house or return home in time to take my vitals. The system was a mobile wireless blue tooth, and I would have to contact my health care provider and advise if the units would be offline for a certain amount of time. Being on this program for four months strengthened my awareness of how my body responded to treatment and if the changes in my life are working. This monitoring system program might not be available through your healthcare provider, but it shouldn't stop you from investing in a good blood pressure machine and a digital scale.

You would be doing yourself an injustice by living with CHF and not monitoring your vitals. Consider when you felt at your worst, you made your way to the ER, and these same procedures for checking vitals took place. When seeing your doctor for a routine visit or being seen in the ER, the first question they ask you is how did you feel when the event occurred, and what do you believe is wrong? The body gives warning signs that you may or may not be aware of when something is not right with your body. With CHF there are noticeable changes within the body, but many people chose to ignore their symptoms. I can't stress enough how important it is to check your vitals daily. At the beginning stages of CHF, the heart is most likely at its weakest. Dealing with the shock of a life-transforming event can be a tough obstacle to overcome. I know for me, monitoring my vitals was the foundation to reversing the effects of CHF in my life. I understand every case may be different for those diagnosed with congestive heart failure as was the case of my father. I've always believed that a healthy mind creates a healthy body. It starts with the will not to give up.

"Wanting something is not enough; you must hunger for it. Your motivation must be absolutely compelling in order to overcome the obstacles that will invariably come your way."
Les Brown.

If you haven't already, I suggest that you invest in a blood pressure monitor, a digital scale and journal your results so that you can accurately monitor your condition. Monitoring my vitals also allowed me to see my body's reaction to certain foods, if my blood pressure medication was working and if I was retaining excess fluids. I don't believe I would have been able to improve my condition without being disciplined in monitoring my vitals.

The Importance of a Low Sodium Diet.
Controlling the amount of sodium in a low salt diet is where so many diagnosed with CHF fail. This is a critical area for a person living with Congestive Heart Failure. A vast majority of CHF patients who are over the age of 40 and are accustomed to a way of eating, making it difficult to change.

You've heard of the old saying, "you can't teach old dogs new tricks." Not only do you have to deal with the shock of being diagnosed with CHF, but you also have to stop eating meals you have been enjoying all of your life and create a healthy eating lifestyle with no time to waste.

At 55 years of age, I lived my entire life enjoying mama's Homestyle soul food cooking, and now all this good eating has to come to an end?

Understanding the importance of a low sodium diet I feel is the blindest area in a CHF patient's life to recovery. When first diagnosed with CFH, your heart is in a weakened state, so the decision to reduce salt and sodium is crucial. When discharged from the hospital, I was provided with a wealth of information on the importance of low sodium diet and guides to eating healthier. The information was very informative, but I felt so disengage from the information because I couldn't at the time see my lifestyle lining up with the guidelines in the pamphlets. Let me better explain; I knew if I followed the instruction of well-researched information, my health would improve. I felt the information didn't understand the culture I lived all my life and in all fairness, how could it? No matter how disconnected I felt from the information I received, I had to make a decision to incorporate this information into my life. In the process of reversing my CHF, the area of controlling sodium was an up and down roller coaster ride. During this time I've learned some serious lesson and had several visits to the ER. Innocently I must say, one time I decided to order a two piece spicy chicken meal from Popeye's Chicken with a side of red beans and rice. Lo and behold, three days later I was back in the ER with breathing problems, fluid overload, and irregular heartbeats. I began to realize this wasn't a game.

So why is controlling sodium so important? With already a weakened heart muscle that's struggling to supply enough blood to the body places pressure on the kidneys which loses its ability to rid the body of salt (sodium) and water. Weakening the kidneys function, causes the body to retain more fluid (pulmonary edema) decreasing the ability to exercise. Fluid may also accumulate in the liver, weakening its capacity to rid the body of toxins and essential proteins. The intestines may become less efficient in absorbing nutrients, and medications and fluid may also accumulate in the extremities resulting in swelling of the ankles and feet. This information was the motivation I needed to reduce my sodium and salt intake and to give my heart a chance to heal.

You owe it to your heart to do your part as it fights to keep your body alive. A major plus in reducing the salt and sodium intake will help lower your blood pressure. I can't stress this enough; you can't start the healing process of CHF without controlling hypertension. Hypertension causes stress on the heart which for many may be the cause of them having congestive heart failure. If you're taking medication to control your blood pressure, continue to remain disciplined to your dosage. Most likely by reducing sodium and being disciplined in taking your medicines, your vital will change. By monitoring your vitals daily, this information will allow your Doctor to make changes to your medications if needed.

I have been challenged with hypertension since college and I've been on blood pressure medication as far as I can remember. I honestly believe years of uncontrolled hypertension contributed to me having CHF. It was very rare that I would have a normal blood pressure reading not realizing the strain it was placing on my heart muscles. Before being introduced to CHF, my blood pressure reading was in the area of 150/95 and a lot of times higher. Two months into a disciplined low sodium diet, my blood pressure reading was in the areas of 120/72 - 130/79. My lower BP reading was a result of reducing my sodium intake to fewer than 2000 mg of sodium per day.

How I approached my low sodium diet. At the beginning stages of CHF, I was instructed to lower my sodium to no more than 1600 mg and no more than 1 ½ liters of water per day. I wasn't aware of how much sodium I was taking in until I started reading the nutritional facts on the back of food labels. There was a time I would enjoy having a can of Nalley's Jalapeno Hot Chili with Beans and some Fritos Corn Chip. Not realizing one can of my favorite chili contain 1130 mg of sodium (2 servings per can), and the Fritos corn chips contained 170 mg of sodium (3 servings per bag.)

Let's do the math. I was placing in my body 2270

mg of sodium and salt in one meal. With a sodium limit of 1600 mg per day, this life change was beginning to look impossible. I now understood why so many don't attempt to take on the challenge to reduce their sodium intake. I started taking closer notice of the nutritional facts on the back of food labels. I knew it was possible to have a low sodium diet but where do you start, there's salt in everything we eat? I didn't realize all of the hidden salts that are in foods such as gravies, instant cereal, package noodles, potato mixes, olives, pickles, soups and canned vegetables are all high in sodium. A good rule of thumb when reading nutritional labels is if the salt or sodium are listed in the first five ingredients, that product is too high in sodium. A lot of shelf herbs and mixed spices are also high in salt. Processed foods have made it so convenient to eat meals quicker while overloading our bodies with unhealthy sodium. So it took some serious commitment on my part to discipline myself to rid my cabinets of all salts and sodium mixed spices. With a wealth of information available to us through the internet, I started researching how to prepare meals that were low in sodium. The information accessible in cyberspace was endless. Great suggestions like cooking with fresh herbs, vinegar, fruit juices, lemon juices and ground pepper added some great flavor. I became so created with cooking that I started preparing dishes I've always enjoyed eating without the salt and very little sodium. Meals like red beans and rice, homemade chili, mustard greens, black-eyed peas, and Popeye's style chicken to name a few. I was now enjoying the foods I was accustomed to eating, now in a healthier way. It was exciting cooking without salt, and my craving for salt in my meals diminished. As much as possible avoid eating frozen processed foods which are very high in sodium. I've always seen frozen foods as frozen fresh, not realizing a lot of frozen meats are soaked in brine or a sodium solution before freezing. A 4oz serving of frozen chicken breast can contain up to 200 – 540 mg of sodium. My favorite frozen item salmon contained up to 910 mg of sodium per serving.

One of the biggest challenges I had to face in this process was what I could and couldn't eat when it came to eating out. Whether it's at a restaurant, a friend's house or a party, it can be difficult if you're serious about your low sodium diet. I noticed that CHF patients approach eating out in one of the three ways. Avoid going out to eat; splurge and don't care about the sodium intake and those who take the time to research healthy places to eat out.

I had an eye-opening experience when it came to eating out at the beginning stages of my CHF. Over a three day period, I ate at In-and-Out burgers, El Pollo Loco and Pizza Hut with my granddaughter. What's was the worry, I've done this many times, and they were small meals. I didn't have a clue of the nutritional facts of the fast foods I was consuming. Five days later my body weight increased by 9 pounds, and I found myself in ER with fluid overload all because of a burger, chicken, and pizza. I couldn't point the blame at the fast foods establishments. When I accepted that I was now living with congestive heart failure, the responsibility was solely on me. I had to make a declaration that I was now eating to live. I was surprised to know that major restaurants and fast food chains have available online or at their establishment nutritional fact sheets. You can view the nutritional facts for many meals you desire to eat. This knowledge made a significant difference in my approach when it came to eating out. For the average American, eating out is convenient and give a nice break from cooking from time to time.

Here are a few tips when deciding to eat out:

- Inform your server that you are on a low sodium diet and ask for suggestions that are low in salt and sodium.

- Order grilled, baked, or boiled meat, chicken, or fish without added salt, sauces, or gravies. Use lemons and peppers to add flavor.
- Select steamed rice, baked potato, or plain noodles instead of mashed potatoes of fried rice.
- If vegetables are not fresh, have a salad instead. Use oil and vinegar dressing or ask for the dressing on the side and use just a bit by dipping.
- Most menu items at fast food restaurants are high in sodium and fats. Ask for the printed nutrition information and choose low sodium options.
- Avoid condiments high in sodium, such as pickles, relish, and olives. Use small amounts of ketchup, mustard, and mayonnaise.

Critical! If your congestive heart failure is alcohol-related, it's especially important that you avoid alcoholic beverages.

HIGH BLOOD PRESSURE AND YOUR HEART

Hypertension (high blood pressure) makes the heart muscles thicken so that it can create more force to pump your blood out. The danger with this, it also injures your arteries making them stiffer and causing your blood pressure to rise even higher. The thicker your heart, the longer it takes to relax. You may start experiencing symptoms like shortness of breath, swelling in your legs, and fatigue. When this occurs it's called Diastolic Heart Failure; when the squeezing portion of the heart remains normal but the relaxing function doesn't.

Controlling your blood pressure is vital to your road to recovery and living a healthier life. As I shared earlier, I believe hypertension played a significant part of the reason I had CHF. Before I could even consider a road to recovery, I had to address controlling my blood pressure. I've been on blood pressure medication as far as I could remember and like so many, we rely on medication to control our blood pressure without any lifestyle changes. It's like placing your body in an internal tug a war, medicine vs. bad habits. So I decided to do some research on a healthier alternative to lowering my blood pressure. I've read several articles stating diets including inorganic nitrates (nitric oxide) can help lower blood pressure. A whole source of inorganic nitrates can be found in soil based plants food, and the most abundant source found in beets.

Beet juice is not only effective in lowering blood pressure, but it also helps to improve the duration and ability to exercise; boost oxygen delivery to the heart while enhanced the general health of the blood vessels. In a small study published in 2010 in the Journal of Applied Physiology, researchers found that adding half a liter of beet juice (also called beetroot juice) to healthy young men's (ages 19 to 38) diets each day improved their exercise performance and duration. Endurance athletes saw a similar benefit from beet juice in another study, published in 2009. And yet another study, published in 2011 in the Journal of Applied Physiology, found that beet juice benefited people ages 54 to 80 who had peripheral vascular disease — a stiffening of the arteries that carry blood to the legs, arms, stomach, or kidneys. I know beet juice played an essential role in my recovery.

In addition to beets, excellent food sources of inorganic nitrates include:
- Cabbage
- Celery

- Chervil
- Chinese cabbage
- Cress
- Dill
- Leek
- Lettuce
- Parsley
- Rucola
- Spinach
- Turnips

By eating these types of inorganic-based food source, they will release nitric oxide into your body.

Two herbs I religiously took that I consider as miracle herbs were garlic and Terminalia Arjuna. Garlic has been used medicinally for at least 3,000 years. Today we are just now discovering what many ancient civilizations including the Romans, Greeks, and Egyptians already knew – garlic boosts strength and prevents disease. It's been said that garlic made Egyptian pyramid-builders stronger and Roman legions more courageous. Garlic contains allicin, one of the most beneficial high blood pressure remedies. A study conducted by researchers from the Russian Academy of Medical Sciences investigated the effects of time-released garlic powder tablets on men with mild to moderate high blood pressure. The research showed that taking a 600 mg time-released garlic tablet decreased blood pressure levels.

It's a known fact; taking garlic regularly can help prevent many chronic health conditions. Studies show garlic is a natural antibacterial and antifungal. It helps with lowering cholesterol naturally and simultaneously acts as a blood thinner. It boosts immunity due to its antioxidant properties, and research has shown it prevents both cancer and cardiovascular disease. It can even treat gastritis. Perhaps one of the most promising actions of this natural "wonder drug" is its ability to lower blood pressure. I use to take once a day what is called, "Garlic Shots." Garlic shot is where you chop up one garlic clove and swallow as if you were taking pills. What I liked about it was you didn't have a garlic taste in your mouth and scent didn't come through your pores.

The second miracle herb that has great benefit is Terminalia Arjuna. Terminalia Arjuna is a huge tree that grows wild in many parts of South Asia, particularly in northern plains of India. The bark of the tree contains natural alkaloids which are very useful Natural care for heart problems. Arjuna (Terminalia Arjuna) bark is beneficial for cardiovascular diseases, congestive heart diseases, high cholesterol, high triglycerides, coronary artery disease, hypertension, etc. Recent research shows that Arjuna is a natural source of CoQ10 (Coenzyme Q10), which is beneficial for strengthening of heart muscles. In my third month with CHF, I started taking Terminalia Arjuna in powder form, mixing with my oatmeal each morning. I begin to notice an improvement in my ability to exercise one month after adding Arjuna to my diet. I honestly believe a great contributor to my health improvement was beet juice, garlic, and Arjuna.

Restoring erectile dysfunction.
I struggled with the thought of having difficulties with erectile dysfunction (ED) and placing myself in an embarrassing situation. Before I could begin to correct this problem, I have to accept the problem of not being able to have a normal erection. If you have heart disease, it's a good chance you have or will have a problem with erectile dysfunction. Like me, many men are reluctant to discuss erectile dysfunction. Sexuality

and a satisfying sexual active life is an important component of quality of life. If there wasn't any other reason to motivate me to make changes to my lifestyle, this was it. If you haven't been diagnosed with having any form of heart disease, but you are experiencing erectile difficulty, it's a good idea to see a qualified healthcare practitioner who can give your heart a thorough check-up. ED could be an early sign of heart disease. Just because you have CHF and currently having difficulties with ED, doesn't mean your sex life is over. NOW, THIS IS GREAT NEWS! As you move in the direction of improving this area, I suggest you seek advice from your doctor or nurse if you're concerned if you should or shouldn't be sexually active.

A healthy green plant diet and exercise can be an asset of improving most health issues when it comes to treating ED. One treatment that is prescribed by many medical physicians for patients with cardiovascular disease is sildenafil (Viagra). Sildenafil success in restoring erectile function is possible in up to 80% of patients. A herb I have found that worked for me was L-arginine. L-arginine is an amino acid naturally present in the body; It helps make nitric oxide. Nitric oxide relaxes blood vessels to facilitate a successful erection. Researchers studied the effects of L=arginine on ED patients. Thirty-one percent of men with Ed taking 5 grams of L=arginine a day experienced significant improvement in sexual function. A Second study showed that L=arginine combined with pycnogenol, a plant product from tree bark, restored the sexual ability to 80 percent of participants after two months. Ninety-two percent had restored sexual ability after three months.

I know firsthand the stress of trying to accept your condition with cardiovascular disease and the embarrassment of having ED. I'm a strong believer that people with CHF can improve in this area and enjoy a quality of life that is not difficult to achieve.

34

CHAPTER 4

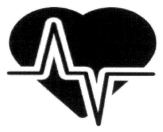

Don't Be Afraid to Exercise

There is almost no disease that exercise doesn't benefit. Just because you had a heart attack, a weak heart (Congestive Heart Failure) or heart disease doesn't mean that you have to sit around and do nothing. In fact, with a regular exercise program, you can hasten your recovery, improve heart function and even get off some of the medication you're on. I'm a living witness to this fact.

A major challenge I faced when it came to exercising, was knowing what my limit was. After being discharged from the hospital, I felt a lot better than when I was first admitted. My blood pressure was under control, I was relieved of excess fluids, and my heart was able to rest. I understood that my heart was recovering from a weakened stage and like any bruised muscle; it needs proper time to heal. I had to keep this in the forefront of my mind as I approached any exercise program. What made it difficult for me was before being diagnosed with CHF, I was accustomed to lifting heavy weights. I now had to approach working out with an entirely new train of thought, resist doing what came naturally for me. Believe me when I say I've learned through trial and error. I didn't start exercising until one week after being discharged from the hospital, and I convinced myself that it would be ok to do half the workout I normally would do. I felt pretty good during my workout, but three hours following working out, I was experiencing some severe irregular heartbeats and dizziness. I guess you can say this was an indication that I overdid it. I waited a few days before working out again, this time I eliminated the free weights and focused on 30 minutes of cardio on the treadmill. 15 minutes into my work out on a low-level pace I decided to increase the incline to the maximum height. After 5 minutes, I begin to experience tightness on my left side of my chest. It felt like there was a 50-pound weight pulling on my chest. No sooner as I stepped off of the treadmill, I was so lightheaded that I had to sit down immediately. I realized early in my recovery I was dealing with an injured muscle and like any good athlete, it was crucial that I give my heart muscle adequate time to heal. I reduced my workout to 15 minutes with light dumbbells, high reps with controlled breathing, followed by 30 minutes of cardio, either on the bicycle or treadmill on medium intensity.

As time progressed, I gradually increased my workout only if I was able to breathe easy during the workout and didn't feel overexerted following my workout. This seemed to work for me, and I gradually started seeing and feeling improvements. Because of my approach toward my diet and exercising, within six months my heart ejection fraction improved from 30% to 55%. In my seventh month, I competed in my first Spartan Sprint race which I was advised by my cardiologist at the beginning stages that it would be at least a year before I could even consider competing in a Spartan Race. A Spartan Sprint consisted of a 5-mile course with a series of 20 + obstacles from fire jump, crawling under barbed wire, slippery walls, tractor tire toss, rope climbs, monkey bars, carrying a bucket full of rocks up a hill and there are hills and hills to run. It took me four hours to complete the course, but I finished, and I felt great about what I've accomplished.

I'm a strong believer that it's never too late to exercise but always check with your doctor first before starting any exercise program for your level of fitness and physical condition.

Dr. Suzanne Steinbaum, a preventive cardiologist at Lenox Hill Hospital in New York City, makes this statement: *"Recommendations to treat heart failure should clearly include an exercise component, heart failure may improve with exercise,"* Steinbaum's study included 60 heart failure patients and 60 healthy people who did either four weeks of supervised aerobic training or no exercise. Half of the participants were 55 and younger, and half were 65 and older. The exercise group undertook four 20-minute training sessions per day, five days a week. They also did one 60-minute group exercise session that focused on muscle endurance and oxygen uptake (a measure of aerobic endurance). Among heart failure patients who exercised, those aged 55 and younger increased their peak oxygen uptake by 25 percent and those aged 65 and older increased it by 27 percent.

According to Steinbaum, those findings demonstrate that **"these beneficial effects of exercise are not age-dependent."**

Lead co-author Dr. Stephan Gielen, Deputy Director of cardiology at the University Hospital, Martin Luther University of Halle, Germany, said in a journal news release. "Exercise switches off the muscle-wasting pathways and switches on pathways involved in muscle growth, counteracting muscle loss and exercise intolerance in heart failure patients," he explained.

I was fortunate to have a nurse practitioner monitor my recovery after being discharged and was able to consult with her whenever I had concerns or questions. Here are some discussion questions I asked:

- How much exercise can I do?
- How often can I exercise each week?
- What type of exercise should I do?
- What kind of activities should I avoid?
- Should I take my medication(s) at a particular time around my exercise schedule?

- Do I have to take my pulse while exercising?

Your doctor may decide to do a stress test or an echocardiogram or modify your medications before starting any exercise program. Always keep your heart's safety in mind. I suggest you start off slow at a lower level. Walking and biking are easy types of workouts for CHF patients. If you haven't been physically active, you should begin your exercise slowly. Your doctor may suggest a workout schedule based on your health condition.

Here is a sample program you may want to try:

- Start with walking or stationary biking for 2 minutes at a comfortable pace. Rest for 1 minute. Repeat this five times, until you have exercised for a total of 10 minutes.

- Over two weeks, gradually increase the exercise period to about 4 minutes and the rest period to 2 minutes, until your total training time is about 20 minutes per session.

- As you become stronger, increase the exercise intervals to 5 minutes and keep the rest intervals to 2 minutes, until your total exercise time is 30 minutes per session. You can also step up your pace.

- Gradually increase the sessions to 40 minutes. You may keep or eliminate the rest stops.
- Vary your program. If you walk for exercise 1 month, for example, try a stationary bike next.

Other exercises your doctor may also prescribe exercises to strengthen muscles. These may include:

- Respiratory muscle exercises to build up your chest, diaphragm, and abdominal muscles to help you breathe better.

- Resistance training that use light weights to strengthen muscle groups in your arms, torso, and legs. Stronger muscles will reduce fatigue.

Done properly, exercise is extremely safe for CHF patients. When you start your training programs, it's a good idea to consult your doctor about how your body is responding. He or she can help you distinguish normal from abnormal responses. A little increase in leg swelling and mild fatigue, for example, are typical during the first few weeks of exercise.

- Be alert for symptoms like chest pain, increasing shortness of breath, weight gain, ankle swelling, abdominal bloating, or rapid pulse at rest. Call your doctor, and stop exercising until the symptoms have diminished.

- Exercise and medication usually work well together. However, if you work out shortly after taking your medicine, you may become dizzy or faint. A change in timing of exercise will often relieve the problem. Also, avoid exercise right after meals.

- Warm up. Before exerting yourself, spend 10 minutes in slow, natural activity— walking slowly and stretching—to increase blood flow to your muscles.

Remember: This information is not intended as a substitute for medical treatment. Before starting an exercise program, consult a physician.

CHAPTER 5

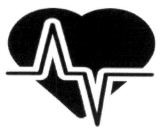

Develop a Healthy Mind and Remain Focused

If you're reading this, CHF is not the end of the world for you although it may appear as such. During my first few weeks of being diagnosed with CHF, I had a lot of questions. My main concern was what is the life expectancy of someone diagnosed with CHF? I was shocked to find out that deaths associated with CHF are 58,824 per years, 4,235 per month, 977 per week, 139 per day and 5 per hour. I witness this first hand with my father who died within the first year with CHF, and this was a major mental obstacle I had to overcome on my road to recovery. Nineteen months after being diagnosed, I'm still here, reversed my CHF and now living a **healthy controlled life. So what made the difference** between my father passing and me living? I don't have the medical knowledge to compare my dad's condition with mine. One difference I am certain of is that my dad gave up. Because of my father's lack of knowledge of his condition, he felt hopeless, failed to make the necessary changes, and allowed fate to run its course. At the time I didn't know how to help my dad, or what to say to encourage him. I watched his need for an oxygen tank, excessive swelling, collapsing, and kidney failure.

Experiencing this, I had to make a decision, so I decided to fight, I decided to live, and I decided to make an effort to see my grandchildren grow up. With the alarming fact that 40% of CHF patients die within the first year forced me to dig deep to find a purpose to fight. I'm a strong believer our minds play an instrumental part in how we view life and respond to life difficulties. A Healthy mind helps create a healthy body. Some of the most amazing stories we've read about people who overcame challenges were individuals who conditioned their minds to accomplish significant achievements. Our minds are our most excellent resource. Proverbs 23:7 tells us, "For as he thinketh in his heart (mind), so is he." Numerous verses in the Bible speak on guarding your mind. Protecting what you allow to go into your thoughts and not allowing negative influences to dictate your thinking.

Rachael Rettner, Senior Writer, in her article, "Heart Disease: Why Positive Attitude May Bring Longer Life," says: "Heart disease patients with a positive attitude live longer than those with a negative attitude, and this boost in survival may be due to increased exercise,"

In her study, heart disease patients with a positive attitude were 42 percent less likely to die over a five-year period than those with a negative attitude. All patients in the study had coronary artery disease or a narrowing or hardening of the arteries that supply blood to the heart. What's more, patients with a positive attitude were about twice as likely to exercise. In fact, further analysis revealed that those with a positive attitude lived longer because they exercised.

Besides exercise, there are multiple reasons why a positive attitude might be good for heart health, said Dr. Suzanne Steinbaum, a preventive cardiologist at Lenox Hill Hospital in New York. Dr. Steinbaum goes on to say; *"A positive outlook may reduce levels of stress hormones and inflammatory markers, and people with a positive outlook tend to adopt other healthier behaviors, such as eating better, sleeping better and not smoking. Individuals who are positive are more likely to do things to take care of themselves, and to help themselves."*

My biggest challenge was to stop focusing on those who died from congestive heart failure and allowing people to tell me about a relative or a friend who died because of CHF. I begin to notice, when I approached people with a sad face, people would respond with a sad face. If I came with a "woos me, I have congestive heart failure," people would respond with, "Oh I'm so sorry to hear you have Congestive Heart Failure." But when I changed my attitude about my condition, it brought about positive responses. I recall a close friend telling me how heartbroken they were to hear that I had congestive heart failure. I responded with, "yes it's true, but I'm doing great, feeling better, and I'm feeling positive about improving my condition." Because of my positive outlook, people would begin to share encouraging stories of family members who are living comfortable lives with CHF for years. I started to google search testimonies of people who were living a healthy fit life with Congestive Heart

Failure. I was so encouraged when I read about an individual who had the same ejection fraction as mine running marathons. Just the excitement I needed to hear which strengthen my focus on reaching my goal. I became so excited about improving my condition that I would be healthy enough to compete in my first Spartan Race. The excitement didn't mean I was walking around with a big silly smile on my face, rather excited about the possibility of what I could accomplish if I applied myself and remain focused. Just as a boxer who is excited about the title fight has on his game face and enters the ring. Their excitement manifested itself in hours of rigorous training and discipline. They're excited about the possibility of achieving their goal and becoming the next world champion. This is the attitude and approach you need to move toward to your recovery. I'll be the first to tell you it's not going always to be peaches and cream especially when you're working through the ups and downs as you find out what works for you.

I remember when I begin working out at the gym, I will listen to motivational speaker Les Brown and Eric Thomas for that extra push.

"Just because fate doesn't deal you the right cards, it doesn't mean you should give up. It means you have to play the cards you get to their maximum potential." Les Brown

I'm a man of faith with a passion and love for God. What brought me the peace I needed to endure what I was about to face was the fact that I knew God was in total control. I believe this was part of a greater plan God had for my life. When it hit me of my condition, depression started to set in. You see, several years prior I went through a divorce of 27 years of marriage. I lost my job and was no longer in full-time ministry. Three areas in my life that was important to me, my pride for my family, career, and ministry. Within a year, all three vanished like a vapor in the wind. Throughout my career, I've never had a problem being employed. Now I found myself unable to find employment anywhere. For the first time in my life, I found myself jobless for eight months. I've worked in the career field of Youth Pastor, Flight Attendant, Youth Counselor, Retail Management and even a Radio Personality. Now I can't find employment? I applied for at least 50 ministry positions and several who did respond back said they were seeking someone with more experience. Wait just a minute; did I miss something here? Did they notice that my resume speaks of 30+ years of ministry experience? Nothing at the time seemed to be working for me, and I endured a difficult period in my life. A year later I was blessed have the job I'm currently working. I vowed two things I will never allow to get out of my control again, my health and my employment. Then came the uninvited guest, Congestive Heart failure. Because the Department of Motor Vehicle (DMV) required a heart ejection fraction of 40% or higher, and my ejection fraction was at 30%, I was no longer qualified to perform my work duties. My employer placed me on administrative leave for eight months while their medical physician reviewed my medical record to determine if I was fit for duty. I didn't realize it at the time, but the time off work was a great opportunity for me to rest, get control of my diet and exercise. I didn't understand the benefits of being off work until it was time for my final health evaluation with my employer. Not only was I surprised by the test results, my cardiologist, and my employers' physician was surprised. I don't have any medical explanation of why, but one thing is for sure, I remained disciplined and stuck to my plan. Being a man of faith, I knew God had the ability to heal me instinctively. I believe God wanted me to do my part, "faith without works is useless." I'm grateful I had the ability to endure what I've been through and wouldn't change what took place if I could. Two great things happened during this time that changed my life. First, God's love for me goes beyond my understanding, getting my attention to take better care of my health. Second, God was also reminding me that He has complete control of my life and if He calls me to take a leap of faith, He's got me, my health and my career.

"God has a purpose for your pain, a reason for your struggles and a reward for your faithfulness, if you don't give up." Eric Thomas

CHAPTER 6

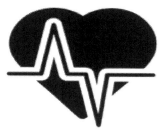

Minimize the Risk as a Commercial Driver

I didn't realize how stressful driving a commercial bus was until I found myself plowing 20 tons of glass and metal through snarled traffic, bikes and jaywalkers. The instant a bus driver sits in the seat, most of the time they are behind schedule, and there's nothing they could do about this. Drivers are prevented from making up time because of traffic congestion, another phenomenon about which they can do nothing about. Further, they are slowed down by passengers insisting on getting on and off the bus. Some passengers may be hostile and abusive, and there's nothing they can do about it. A schedule rules your life as a bus operator, not eating the right foods, drink enough water or even relieve yourself when you should. There's no such thing as a lunch or bathroom break while sitting all day in an isolated driver's area. If you have the personality like mines, you'll find yourself engaged in conversations with people all day. By the time I pulled my 20-ton bus back into the yard at the end of my shift, I'm exhausted. Commercial driving indeed can provide a decent living, but it can also lead to a short life.

Research has found that workers who have little control over work pace and methods, experience higher levels of catecholamines, epinephrine (adrenaline) leading to mental strain and coronary disease. It's no wonder why the transportation industry is experiencing high absenteeism amongst drivers who are trying to escape the stress that comes with the job.

Christine Zook, former president of Amalgamated Transit Union Local 192, said; "the fact of the matter is, we die young. The job will kill you over time." Bus drivers are among the unhealthiest of occupational groups, especially about cardiovascular, gastrointestinal and musculoskeletal disorder according to the Journal of Occupational Health, Psychology in 1998. Numerous studies show that cardiovascular mortality rate is directly linked to years of service as a driver. Commercial bus operators are also prone to increased blood pressure and high levels of stress hormones which contribute to sickness and death from heart and blood vessel problems.

I recall my employer's medical physician expressing his concern if I was healthy enough to remain in the career field as a bus driver even if I show improvement. With his extensive knowledge of the industries health challenges, he suggested that I look into a career field that would be less stressful. After six months being on administrative leave, my condition did improve, and I was reinstated back to my position as a bus driver. Now I was faced with this question, "how do I prevent this from ever happening again?" While I was out on administrative leave, it was a lot simpler to maintain a healthy lifestyle. Being back in the driver's seat, I don't have nearly the flexibility.

Working in transportation, you quickly learn the importance of keeping a schedule. So much, that a lot of operators experience stress and anxiety if they're not able to maintain their schedule. I was one of those drivers, and I couldn't afford to repeat what took place with my health, so I had to return to work with an entirely different mindset. The biggest challenge so many drivers and I face as we approach our work day is how do we minimize the risk?

When you have so many uncertainties in your workday as a commercial driver, it seems almost impossible to reduce the risks. Faced with this dilemma, you only have two options, except the harsh condition and hope for the best, or make a conscious decision to initiate a plan to minimize the health risk in your workday.

There are four basic, easy controllable activities a driver can take to minimize their risk:

1. Take care of your body and mind.
Encompass a combination of diet, exercise, and rest. I believe a healthy nutritional diet is the foundation to your road to a healthier lifestyle. Here are some healthy eating tips when it comes to packing your lunch for the work day:

- Cauliflower florets
- Broccoli florets

- Baby carrots
- Snap peas
- Edamame
- Celery sticks
- Sliced mangos
- Cherries
- Apples
- Dried fruit
- Grapes
- Squeezable applesauce
- Salads in a jar

If you aren't a fan of veggies straight up, you can also pack some dipping sauce.

Great source of protein that will keep you from being hungry and eating all are:

- Yogurt; (Look for higher fat versions with less sugar or make your own.)
- Jerky; (There are lots of healthier version without additives.)
- Grilled chicken sandwich
- Almonds
- Cheese
- Hard-boiled eggs
- Roasted chickpeas

- Cheese crackers; tasty, and surprisingly high in protein!
- Nut butter packets; it's like a shot of liquid energy
- Energy bars; pick up your favorites, or make some granola bars or date bites at home before you leave
- Hummus
- Sweet Treats
- Graham crackers
- Animal crackers
- Whole grain cookies
- Dark chocolate
- Chocolate covered fruit or nuts

Ditch the boxes and bags on most items; you can do some serious condensing if you leave at home the packaging it came it. Pull everything out and repackage what needs to be repackaged in smaller, stackable containers. Head to the dollar store and pick up an open tote to hold your non-refrigerated snacks. That way everything is readily available and easy to see.

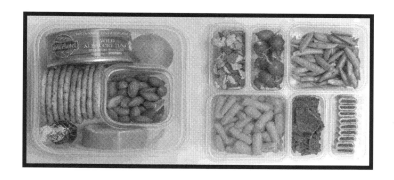

2. Identify your priorities and establish boundaries.

Consider what is most important and valuable to you during your workday. For example; exercising and controlling stress is a high priority for me, required me to set boundaries around these priorities. Because exercising was a priority I had to set boundaries to ensure that I was able to get to the gym either before work, during a split or after work.

3. Be realistic and don't beat yourself down.

Assess your expectations of your goals with others drivers who are like minded. It's good to build a support group that will help each other be accountable. Try not to expect fast instant results and don't become discouraged if you fall off the track at times. Realize it's not about being perfect,

rather making an effort to live a healthy lifestyle.
I understand in this profession conflicts will arise unexpectedly. So I don't approach my workday with the expectation that my goals may not go according to plans. Instead, I plan ahead for healthy responses to conflicts that may arise and be prepared to set more boundaries if needed.

4. Cultivate gratitude.

There is growing research on the benefits of gratitude, particularly on physical, psychological, and relational well-being. Dr. Robert Emmons, a leading researcher on the Science of Gratitude, calls it; "attitude of gratitude." Gratitude has been linked to greater stress tolerance, increased positive emotions, better sleep, improved physical health, and healthier relationships. It can be beneficial to create a daily habit of remembering what you are thankful for. Keeping a gratitude list at the beginning or end of each day is an excellent way to do this. If certain well-meaning friends or family members start stretching your patience, remind yourself of why you are thankful to have them in your life. As a bus operator, I witness a lot of poverty, homelessness, and people less fortunate than me. I recall a young lady riding my bus for hours to get her six months and two year-old babies out of the scourging heat because they were homeless. There's not a driver who hasn't witness individuals who are less fortunate than them. With an attitude of appreciative and gratefulness, it will help you to respond to people and stress differently.

"Perseverance is the hard work you do after you get tired of doing the hard work you already did." Newt Gingrich

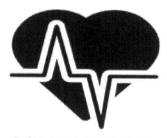

CONCLUSION

The leading cause of death in America is not heart diseases, cancer, stroke or diabetes. More than 70 percent of adults across the United States have been diagnosed with choric illness. More than 75 percent of the national healthcare cost is spent on managing and treating these conditions. **The greatest cause of death is the mindset to do nothing about your situation.** I can't tell you how many people I have come in contact with who are living with CHF but made no attempts at making changes and my father being one of those persons. When it comes to your health, I don't believe it fair for a patient to place all of the responsibility for their wellness upon the medical physician. Sadly, so many do every day.

Study shows less than 3 percent of Americans live a healthy lifestyle, while the remaining 97 percent of Americans live an unhealthy way of life. What's even more disturbing, more than half of what Americans eat is "ultra-processed," meaning that they have been processed so much that they are no longer recognized as plants. It's no secret that the foods we consume are sending us to an early grave. I've shared earlier in this book the benefits of exercising. Exercising without a doubt is one of the most powerful ways to improve your health condition. Regular exercising can reduce the risks and symptoms of more than 20 physical and mental health conditions, and can slow down how quickly your body ages. A healthy diet along with exercising is the greatest combination you can do to improve your health.

Don't label your condition for failure. You have more control over your health than you think. You're the one in control! Manage, and you can avoid 60 -70 percent of known chronic conditions with exercise, nutrition, and mental balance.

You Can Beat This!

"Champions aren't made in gyms. Champions are made from something they have deep inside them-a desire, a dream, a vision. They have to have the skill and the will. But the will must be stronger than the skill."

Muhammad Ali

Low Sodium Recipes

For video tutorials visit Westbrooks Kitchen YOUTUBE page.

Spicy Stuffed Bell Peppers

Ingredients:
6 Bell whole bell peppers
1 LB of ground turkey
½ cup mozzarella cheese
¾ cups of cooked rice
½ of parmesan cheese
2 tablespoons of cilantro
1 ½ cups of marinara sauce
2 tablespoons of olive oil
2 ounces of cream cheese
1 pack Mrs. Dash low sodium taco seasoning
½ cup of celery
½ cup of green onions
¼ cup of water

Slice the tops of each pepper. (I like using different color peppers, gives a better presentation.) Clean out all seeds out of peppers. In a heated skillet add in 2 tbsp. of olive oil. Add in chopped onions and celery and Sautee until tender. Add ground turkey and drain any fats if any. Add Mrs. Dash taco seasoning. Add in marinara sauce, rice, cream cheese, parmesan cheese, cilantro, and stir and mix well. Bring to a light boil and allow cool. Fill each pepper with meat filling and place in a roasting pan. After all, peppers are placed in the roasting pan, sprinkle mozzarella cheese on top of the peppers. Pour into the pan ¼ cup of water which will keep the peppers from sticking and allow steam. In a preheated oven on 375, cook for 30, to 35 minutes.

Low Sodom Black Eye Peas

Ingredients:
1 LB of ground turkey (beef)
1 onion
3 Garlic Cloves
½ cup of green bell pepper
½ cup of red bell pepper
3 chopped jalapeno
½ teaspoon Cummins
½ teaspoon cayenne pepper
1 teaspoon black pepper
1 teaspoon Tony Chachere's Cajun
  seasoning
½ teaspoon Silvia's secret seasoning
½ teaspoon Tony Chachere's salt-free
  seasoning.

Cook meat and drain any fat. In your slow cooker, pour in water and broth. Place in ground meat, beans, onions, garlic, peppers, jalapenos, and all seasoning. Give it a good stir and cook for 4 hours on high or 8 hours on low. ENJOY!

Blackened Red Snapper

Ingredients:

Fresh Snapper or Rockfish

Rub: ½ teaspoon of South African smoke seasoning (Trader Joes)

½ teaspoon Tony Chachere's Cajun seasoning

1 teaspoon of themes

¼ cayenne peppers

¼ teaspoon smoked paprika

½ teaspoon oregano

½ teaspoon onion powder

½ teaspoon garlic powder

1 teaspoon black pepper

½ teaspoon lemon pepper

With a napkin, dry pieces of fish. Using your hands place olive oil on both sides of each piece. Massage rub on both sides of each piece of fish. In a preheated skillet, pour in 1 tablespoon of olive oil in the skillet. Depending on skillet size, cook a few pieces at a time evenly separated. Depending on the thickness of your fish, cook on each side for four minutes each. To add a little more flavor, place small pieces of unsalted butter around fish as they cook. Cook until your fish has a nice blackened texture.

Stuffed Spinach & Crab Mushrooms

Ingredients:

16 Small Portobello mushrooms

4 oz crab meat. (Spouts has refrigerated crab meat with less sodium)

16 oz of baby spinach

4 oz cream cheese

½ cup mozzarella cheese

3 eggs

3 tablespoon olive oil

3 chopped garlic cloves

2 chopped jalapeno

½ teaspoon Silvia's secret seasoning

½ teaspoon of salt-free lemon pepper

Clean each mushroom and with a spoon scrape out the inner body. In a heated saucepan, pour in three tablespoons of olive oil. Add the garlic, chopped jalapeno, and seasonings. Add in spinach and cook down. Allow to cool and chop the spinach into smaller pieces because we're using smaller mushrooms. If you decide to use larger mushrooms, you can leave as is. In a mixing bowl mix in spinach, mozzarella cheese, cream cheese, eggs, crab meat and mix well. Stuff each mushroom with ingredients and place on a cooking sheet. Spray cooking sheet with non-stick to prevent mushrooms from sticking. Place in a preheated oven at 375 for 20 minutes.

Slow Cooker Falling off the Bone Baby Backs Ribs

Ingredients:
2 slabs of baby back ribs
1 sliced onion
1 slice green bell pepper
1 cup of beer (optional)
¼ cup of barbecue sauce
Mustard
Liquid smoke
Lemon juice
Zesty table blend seasoning (use low-sodium spice seasonings you enjoy.)
Trader Joes 12 salute seasoning
Trader Joes South African Rub (or Cajun seasoning.)
Low sodium lemon pepper
Silvia's secret seasoning

Clean your ribs by cutting off excess fats. Because we're placing our ribs in a slow cooker, it's best to cut each slab into two pieces. With your hands massage your ribs with yellow mustard, liquid smoke, and lemon juice. Evenly add all seasoning to both sides of your ribs and do a soft rub. Place ribs in slow cooker upright and place onions and peppers surrounding the ribs. Pour in beer and 1 tablespoon of liquid smoke, ¼ cup of barbecue sauce. Cook in slow cooker on high for 4 hours. After four hours in slow cooker place ribs in a preheated conventional oven on 375 for 15 minutes. Option: add more barbecue sauce prior to placing in the oven.

Salisbury Steak

Ingredients:
1 ½ LB ground beef
½ cup French onion soup (Low sodium, Trader Joes)
½ cup breadcrumbs
1 egg
½ tsp. Salt-free seasoning
¼ tsp. Black pepper
1 tbsp. all-purpose flour
½ cup catchup
1 tbsp. Worchester sauce
½ tsp mustard powder
¼ cup red wine (optional)

In a large mixing bowl, place in ground beef, French onion soup, bread crumbs, egg, all seasonings, squeeze and mix. Shape beef into oval patties and in a preheated skillet lightly oiled, brown both sides of beef patties. (While the patties are browning.) In a separate bowl, add in flour, mustard powder, catchup, red wine, Worchester sauce, sliced mushrooms and remaining French onion soup. Pour over patties and cook covered for 25 minutes.

Spicy Jamaican Jerk Hot Wings

Ingredients:
3 to 4 LB hot wings
½ cup Onion,
3 Garlic Cloves
½ cup Green onion
4 Habanero peppers
1 tablespoon Thyme
1 tsp Salt Tony Chachere's salt-free seasoning
1 tsp Black pepper
1 ½ tablespoon Allspice
½ tsp Cinnamon
½ tsp Ground Cummins
½ tsp Nutmeg
½ tsp Cajun seasoning
1 ½ tbsp. Vegetable oil
1 tbsp. Brown sugar
1 ½ tbsp. Lime juice
1 ½ tbsp. Liquid smoke
(Optional) ¼ cup of low sodium soy sauce88

Place all of your ingredients in a blender and blend to a fine texture. You want to blend it course enough to use as a marinade. Place your chicken in a bowl and completely cover with your marinade. Cover and refrigerate overnight or for 8 hours. Spray a cooking sheet with a nonstick and place hot wings evenly on cooking sheet. Save the extra marinade we're going to use it later to add extra marinade during the cooking process. Place hot wings in a preheated oven on 400 and cook for 25 minutes. Remove hot wings from the over and with a brush add another layer of marinade on both sides your wings. Place back in the oven for 10 minutes and repeat marinade process. You want to do this for a period of 3 times.

Slow Cooker Spicy Mustard Greens with Kale

Ingredients:

5 bunches of Chinese mustard greens

3 bunches of Kale

5 chopped jalapeno

3 Garlic Cloves

1 green bell pepper

1 red bell pepper

2 Tablespoons olive oil

2 2 tablespoons balsamic vinegar

1 tablespoon liquid smoke

16 oz low sodium chicken broth (Trader Joes)

1 onion

½ tablespoon Silvia's secret seasoning

½ Tony Chachere's salt-free seasoning

¼ tablespoon black pepper

¼ smoked paprika

1 tables spoon Trader Joes 12 salute seasoning

½ tablespoon Trader Joes South African Rub (or Cajun seasoning.)

½ tsp ground red pepper

½ tablespoon lemon pepper

In a preheated skillet, add in olive oil, liquid smoke, vinegar, chopped garlic, onions, jalapeno, and Sautee. In a large pot, pour in chicken broth, Sautee vegetable and bring to a boil. Add in your greens and kale and cook down. After greens and kale have cooked down for 10 minutes, pour into your slow cooker and add in all of your seasonings. Cook on high for 4 hours or low for 8 hours.

Life Vital Chart

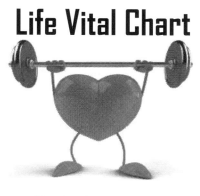

Daily Log Sheet

Date:	Blood Pressure Reading	Weight	Symptoms

Did you exercise today? _____Yes _____ No

Log workout:

Date:	Blood Pressure Reading	Weight	Symptoms

Did you exercise today? _____Yes _____ No

Log workout:

Date:	Blood Pressure Reading	Weight	Symptoms

Did you exercise today? _____Yes _____ No

Log workout:

Date:	Blood Pressure Reading	Weight	Symptoms

Did you exercise today? _____Yes _____ No

Log workout:

Date:	Blood Pressure Reading	Weight	Symptoms
Did you exercise today? ____Yes ____ No			

Log workout:

Date:	Blood Pressure Reading	Weight	Symptoms
Did you exercise today? ____Yes ____ No			

Log workout:

Date:	Blood Pressure Reading	Weight	Symptoms
Did you exercise today? ____Yes ____ No			

Log workout:

Date:	Blood Pressure Reading	Weight	Symptoms
Did you exercise today? ____Yes ____ No			

Log workout:

Date:	Blood Pressure Reading	Weight	Symptoms

Did you exercise today? _____ Yes _____ No

Log workout:

Date:	Blood Pressure Reading	Weight	Symptoms

Did you exercise today? _____ Yes _____ No

Log workout:

Date:	Blood Pressure Reading	Weight	Symptoms

Did you exercise today? _____ Yes _____ No

Log workout:

Date:	Blood Pressure Reading	Weight	Symptoms

Did you exercise today? _____ Yes _____ No

Log workout:

Date:	Blood Pressure Reading	Weight	Symptoms
Did you exercise today? _____ Yes _____ No			

Log workout:

Date:	Blood Pressure Reading	Weight	Symptoms
Did you exercise today? _____ Yes _____ No			

Log workout:

Date:	Blood Pressure Reading	Weight	Symptoms
Did you exercise today? _____ Yes _____ No			

Log workout:

Date:	Blood Pressure Reading	Weight	Symptoms
Did you exercise today? _____ Yes _____ No			

Log workout:

Date:	Blood Pressure Reading	Weight	Symptoms

Did you exercise today? _____Yes _____ No

Log workout:

Date:	Blood Pressure Reading	Weight	Symptoms

Did you exercise today? _____Yes _____ No

Log workout:

Date:	Blood Pressure Reading	Weight	Symptoms

Did you exercise today? _____Yes _____ No

Log workout:

Date:	Blood Pressure Reading	Weight	Symptoms

Did you exercise today? _____Yes _____ No

Log workout:

Date:	Blood Pressure Reading	Weight	Symptoms

Did you exercise today? _____Yes _____ No

Log workout:

Date:	Blood Pressure Reading	Weight	Symptoms

Did you exercise today? _____Yes _____ No

Log workout:

Date:	Blood Pressure Reading	Weight	Symptoms

Did you exercise today? _____Yes _____ No

Log workout:

Date:	Blood Pressure Reading	Weight	Symptoms

Did you exercise today? _____Yes _____ No

Log workout:

Date:	Blood Pressure Reading	Weight	Symptoms

Did you exercise today? _____ Yes _____ No

Log workout:

Date:	Blood Pressure Reading	Weight	Symptoms

Did you exercise today? _____ Yes _____ No

Log workout:

Date:	Blood Pressure Reading	Weight	Symptoms

Did you exercise today? _____ Yes _____ No

Log workout:

Date:	Blood Pressure Reading	Weight	Symptoms

Did you exercise today? _____ Yes _____ No

Log workout:

Date:	Blood Pressure Reading	Weight	Symptoms

Did you exercise today? _____ Yes _____ No

Log workout:

Date:	Blood Pressure Reading	Weight	Symptoms

Did you exercise today? _____ Yes _____ No

Log workout:

Date:	Blood Pressure Reading	Weight	Symptoms

Did you exercise today? _____ Yes _____ No

Log workout:

Date:	Blood Pressure Reading	Weight	Symptoms

Did you exercise today? _____ Yes _____ No

Log workout:

Date:	Blood Pressure Reading	Weight	Symptoms

Did you exercise today? _____ Yes _____ No

Log workout:

Date:	Blood Pressure Reading	Weight	Symptoms

Did you exercise today? _____ Yes _____ No

Log workout:

Date:	Blood Pressure Reading	Weight	Symptoms

Did you exercise today? _____ Yes _____ No

Log workout:

Date:	Blood Pressure Reading	Weight	Symptoms

Did you exercise today? _____ Yes _____ No

Log workout:

Date:	Blood Pressure Reading	Weight	Symptoms

Did you exercise today? ____ Yes ____ No

Log workout:

Date:	Blood Pressure Reading	Weight	Symptoms

Did you exercise today? ____ Yes ____ No

Log workout:

Date:	Blood Pressure Reading	Weight	Symptoms

Did you exercise today? ____ Yes ____ No

Log workout:

Date:	Blood Pressure Reading	Weight	Symptoms

Did you exercise today? ____ Yes ____ No

Log workout:

Date:	Blood Pressure Reading	Weight	Symptoms

Did you exercise today? _____ Yes _____ No

Log workout:

Date:	Blood Pressure Reading	Weight	Symptoms

Did you exercise today? _____ Yes _____ No

Log workout:

Date:	Blood Pressure Reading	Weight	Symptoms

Did you exercise today? _____ Yes _____ No

Log workout:

Date:	Blood Pressure Reading	Weight	Symptoms

Did you exercise today? _____ Yes _____ No

Log workout:

Date:	Blood Pressure Reading	Weight	Symptoms

Did you exercise today? _____ Yes _____ No

Log workout:

Date:	Blood Pressure Reading	Weight	Symptoms

Did you exercise today? _____ Yes _____ No

Log workout:

Date:	Blood Pressure Reading	Weight	Symptoms

Did you exercise today? _____ Yes _____ No

Log workout:

Date:	Blood Pressure Reading	Weight	Symptoms

Did you exercise today? _____ Yes _____ No

Log workout:

Date:	Blood Pressure Reading	Weight	Symptoms
Did you exercise today? _____Yes _____ No			

Log workout:

Date:	Blood Pressure Reading	Weight	Symptoms
Did you exercise today? _____Yes _____ No			

Log workout:

Date:	Blood Pressure Reading	Weight	Symptoms
Did you exercise today? _____Yes _____ No			

Log workout:

Date:	Blood Pressure Reading	Weight	Symptoms
Did you exercise today? _____Yes _____ No			

Log workout:

Date:	Blood Pressure Reading	Weight	Symptoms

Did you exercise today? _____Yes _____ No

Log workout:

Date:	Blood Pressure Reading	Weight	Symptoms

Did you exercise today? _____Yes _____ No

Log workout:

Date:	Blood Pressure Reading	Weight	Symptoms

Did you exercise today? _____Yes _____ No

Log workout:

Date:	Blood Pressure Reading	Weight	Symptoms

Did you exercise today? _____Yes _____ No

Log workout:

Date:	Blood Pressure Reading	Weight	Symptoms

Did you exercise today? ____Yes ____ No

Log workout:

Date:	Blood Pressure Reading	Weight	Symptoms

Did you exercise today? ____Yes ____ No

Log workout:

Date:	Blood Pressure Reading	Weight	Symptoms

Did you exercise today? ____Yes ____ No

Log workout:

Date:	Blood Pressure Reading	Weight	Symptoms

Did you exercise today? ____Yes ____ No

Log workout:

Date:	Blood Pressure Reading	Weight	Symptoms

Did you exercise today? _____ Yes _____ No

Log workout:

Date:	Blood Pressure Reading	Weight	Symptoms

Did you exercise today? _____ Yes _____ No

Log workout:

Date:	Blood Pressure Reading	Weight	Symptoms

Did you exercise today? _____ Yes _____ No

Log workout:

Date:	Blood Pressure Reading	Weight	Symptoms

Did you exercise today? _____ Yes _____ No

Log workout: